Contents

Y0-BSS-973

NOTE: The course you take may contain information on CPR for infants or children or both. Check with your instructor to find out which sections of the book you should study.

Written material alone does not constitute a CPR course. To gain the skills of CPR, it is necessary to practice with manikins, with trained instructors as guides.

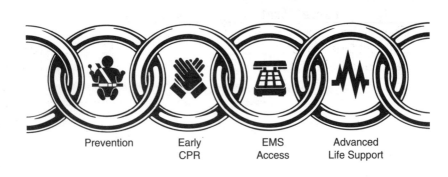

Prevention   Early   EMS   Advanced
             CPR   Access   Life Support

Introduction

Injuries are one of the leading causes of death and disability in children. One of every three deaths among children in the United States results from an injury. The total number of injuries, of course, far exceeds the number of deaths.

This year one of five children will have an injury serious enough to require treatment in a hospital emergency room. That is one of five children in your neighborhood, one of five in your family, one of five in your care, and this statistic does not include visits to the doctor's office or treatment at home.

Injuries can cause a moment's fright, a wave of guilt, and a few hours or days of healing. They can also cause serious brain and other organ damage, long-term disability, incredible anguish, and even death.

Injuries to children occur everywhere. They occur in cities, suburbs, and rural areas; in high-, middle-, and low-income families; in large apartment buildings and single-family homes; in schools and day-care centers; on streets and playgrounds; and in cars.

The goal of this course is to reduce the number of childhood deaths caused by injuries and breathing or cardiovascular problems. This can be accomplished in part by reducing hazards in the child's environment and promoting safe practices in everyday living. To do this, parents and caregivers need to know how children are injured and how those injuries can be prevented. The safety section of this course provides that information. The goal of the course can also be accomplished by teaching emergency measures to clear the airway and perform cardiopulmonary resuscitation (CPR).

At the heart of the program is the checklist in Appendix B. It serves as a guide for an inspection of your home, school, day-care facility, or wherever a child spends time. By following the recommendations you can help create a safe environment and reduce the chance of injury.

It is beyond the scope of this or any course or book to alert you to every hazard in a child's environment. For this reason, young children must not be left unsupervised. While it is up to you to watch them carefully, caring for children can be made easier by creating an environment that is as free of hazards as possible.

The American Academy of Pediatrics (AAP) offers additional information on injury prevention. The Injury Prevention Program (TIPP) was developed by the AAP to help physicians teach parents how to help their children avoid injuries. Ask your doctor about The Injury Prevention Program.

Unfortunately children do get hurt, even in safe environments. The extent of injury can be minimized and death may even be prevented by the actions of a trained caregiver. In this course you will learn how to perform CPR and how to give first aid to infants and children who are choking.

These skills can help save lives. As you learn the steps of basic lifesaving you will learn how to

- Recognize an infant or child in distress
- Act quickly and effectively to get help
- Help a choking infant or child by performing the correct maneuvers for relief of foreign-body airway obstruction (FBAO)
- Activate the emergency medical services (EMS) system
- Help an infant or child who is not breathing or is without a heartbeat by performing CPR

The course has two sessions, each lasting approximately 3 or 4 hours (depending on whether your course teaches procedures for infants or children or both). The following topics will be covered:

Session 1
Welcome and introduction of instructors
Program overview
Infant and child safety
CPR for infants and/or children
Relief of FBAO in infants and/or children

Session 2
Review of safety inspection using the checklist
Review of CPR and techniques for relieving FBAO
Written examination
Evaluation of CPR
Evaluation of techniques for relieving FBAO

Some rescue procedures are performed in the same way regardless of the victim's age. A few procedures are performed differently, depending on whether the victim is an infant (under 1 year old) or a child (1 to 8 years old). Because of time limitations, the course you are taking may emphasize the procedures for one age group. If this is the case, you will be evaluated on only the procedures taught. This course does not teach the techniques of CPR and relief of FBAO for children older than 8 years and for adult victims. Such techniques differ from those for infants and children, and are described in other American Heart Association (AHA) textbooks (eg, *Heartsaver Guide*). If you want to learn more, ask your instructor about additional courses.

Adults must make the environments of young children as safe as possible and must care for children in case of an injury. Anyone who cares for young children can benefit from this program. You can create and maintain safe places for children to live and play. You can save lives by preventing injuries and performing the correct maneuvers when a child is hurt or has difficulty breathing.

By taking this course, you will take a big step toward reducing childhood injuries and deaths. Your hard work and study can make a difference.

1
The Emergency Medical Services System

An EMS system is a communitywide, coordinated means of responding to sudden illness or injury. It is a complete rescue system. An effective EMS system has many elements. You must understand two of these:

- Entry into the system
- Rescue and transportation

Entry Into the System

Everyone should be able to recognize the warning signals of choking and breathing difficulty in patients of all ages, as well as the signals of heart attack and stroke in adults. Everyone should be able to provide immediate emergency care to sustain life until arrival of EMS personnel.

As soon as an emergency is recognized, a bystander or some delegated person must place a telephone call to activate the EMS system. If the emergency involves a child, however, a trained rescuer should begin CPR *immediately* and send someone else to activate the EMS system. When telephoning for help, be prepared to provide the following information:

1. *Where* the emergency is, giving the address or names of cross streets, roads, or other landmarks if possible
2. *Telephone number* from which you are calling
3. *What happened* — auto accident, fall, breathing difficulty, etc
4. *How many* persons need help
5. *Condition* of the victim(s)
6. *What* is being done for the victim(s)
7. *Any other* information requested

Hang up only when told to do so by the operator/dispatcher.

Rescue and Transportation

Bystanders trained in basic life support should perform immediate rescue procedures, including CPR when indicated, until the EMS system or local rescue unit responds. When trained professionals arrive at the scene, they assume responsibility for the victim.

If an EMS system is not available in your community, the victim should be taken immediately to the nearest hospital emergency department.

Know your local emergency telephone number and keep it posted near your telephone. (In many communities this is 911. If you are not sure, check your telephone book.)

Know the location of the nearest emergency department that can provide 24-hour emergency care.

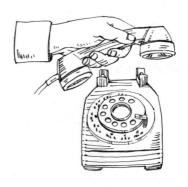

2
Infant and Child Safety

The most common causes of fatal injuries in infants, children, and adolescents include motor vehicle crashes, pedestrian or bicycle-related head injuries, burns or smoke inhalation, falls, firearms (including unintentional injuries, homicides, and suicides), and drowning. Many of these injuries can be avoided if we are aware of the hazards around our children and if we take steps to reduce these hazards. We must do this in our homes, schools, day-care centers, and wherever our children spend time. We must promote safe practices in everyday living.

We must also be aware that young children cannot care for themselves. If left alone, they may get hurt. As adults who care for young children, we must always be aware of our responsibilities, which vary according to the ages of the children. No environment is totally safe. The most important element in any child-safety program may well be a watchful and attentive adult.

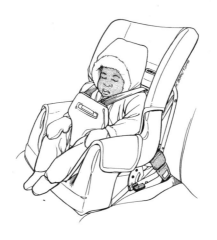

Motor Vehicle and Traffic Safety

Injuries suffered while riding in cars are the No. 1 preventable cause of death in young children.

Young children are easily thrown in an impact. Because a young child's head is large in proportion to the body, unrestrained children tend to fly head-first into the windshield or head-first out of the car when a collision occurs. Severe or fatal head injuries often result. Even in a low-speed crash, an infant or small child can smash into the windshield, dashboard, or air bag with a force comparable to falling from a third-story window. It is not safe to hold a child on your lap in a car. In the event of a crash, the child will be thrown into the body of the car or be crushed by your weight.

The BACK seat is the BEST seat for children 12 years old or younger. In this location in the automobile, the properly restrained child is least likely to sustain injuries in a crash because the child is away from the dashboard and windshield and is prevented from being catapulted out of the seat.

You have probably heard about injuries resulting from air bags. Air bags are designed to save lives when used with seat belts and they can protect drivers and passengers who are correctly "buckled up." An air bag inflates very quickly and forcefully to cushion a victim during a crash. When it inflates, an air bag can strike anything or anyone — including children — located too near the dashboard, and the impact of the air bag can cause serious head and neck injuries. Air bags have saved more than 1500 lives nationwide, but air bag deployment also has been associated with the deaths of several children and a small adult. Most of those injured by air bags have *not* used car seats and seat belts properly.

No infants or children in car seats should be positioned in the front seat of a car with a passenger-side air bag. Rear-facing infant seats should **never** be secured in the front seat of any car with a passenger-side air bag. A rear-facing safety seat positions the infant's head very near the front of the car, near the dashboard. If the air bag inflates, it can drive the infant seat into the back of the automobile seat, injuring the infant's head and neck. In a car seat even a child aged 1 to 4 years may be injured by an air bag because the car seat positions the child near the front of the automobile seat, close to the dashboard and the air bag. Until "smart" air bags are widely available, the following steps can reduce the risk of injury from air bags:

- All car passengers must be properly restrained in seat belts.
  - *Infants less than 20 pounds or under 1 year:* Use rear-facing car seats in the BACK seat. **Never** place an infant in the front seat of a car with a passenger-side air bag.
  - *Infants more than 20 pounds and children up to 4 years old:* Use car seats in the BACK seat.
- Children over 4 years old and adults: Use lap and shoulder belts. Be sure that the lap belt rests low across the child's hips and that the shoulder belt crosses from hip to shoulder, not across the neck. Child safety seats may be needed for children 4 to 7 years old to restrain them properly with a lap-shoulder restraint system.
- The BEST seat for children 12 years old and younger is the BACK seat.
  - **Never** place an infant in the front seat of a car with a passenger-side air bag.
  - **No** children in car seats should be in the front seat.
  - If possible, only adults and children over 12 years old should sit in the front seat.
- When children or small adults are seated in the front seat, move the front seat as far away from the dashboard as possible.
- For questions about children and air bags, call the National Highway Traffic Safety Administration Auto Safety Hotline toll-free at 1-800-424-9393.

Car safety seats and seat belts can prevent most severe injuries to passengers of all ages if they are used correctly. Infants and children up to 4 years of age or 40 pounds in weight must always ride in a car safety seat. The safety seat will hold the child securely in the car and help absorb the forces of even violent crashes. The child must be secured in the car safety seat with the harness or straps that are part of the safety seat, and the safety seat must also be secured in the car using the car seat belt. The car safety seat should be secured in the back seat of the car, particularly if the car has a passenger-side air bag.

Children older than 4 years or larger than 40 pounds in weight should always wear seat restraints when riding in cars. Lap and shoulder belts provide better protection than lap belts alone. The shoulder belt should cross from the child's shoulder across the chest to the hips. The lap belt should be adjusted until it is snug, and it should rest over the child's hips. All children 12 years old and younger should be restrained in the back seat of the car. If it is necessary to carpool children in a car with a passenger-side air bag, put the largest child in the front seat (no children in car safety seats) and move the seat as far away from the dashboard as possible.

Children learn by example. Be sure that you — and every person who rides with you — are buckled up for *every* ride. Follow the watchwords of the AAP and "Make every ride a safe ride." Remember, the BEST seat for children 12 years old and younger is the BACK seat.

Not all children who die from traffic injuries are passengers in cars. Many are injured while walking or playing near streets or while riding bicycles. Infants and toddlers are most commonly injured by cars backing up in driveways or parking lots. Children between the ages of 5 and 9 who are struck by cars typically dart out in front of traffic in the middle of the block. Parents must supervise children closely; adults must watch for children when driving. Children must be taught early in life to cross streets at intersections, to always stop at curbs, and to *stop, look* both ways, and *listen* for cars before crossing any street.

Children riding bicycles can be injured when they collide with cars or other fixed objects or when they are thrown from the bicycle. The most serious bicycle-related injuries are head injuries, which can cause death or permanent brain damage. Most (85%) of these head injuries can be prevented if children wear bicycle helmets approved by the Snell Memorial Foundation or the American National Standards Institute (ANSI) *whenever* they ride a bicycle. The helmet must fit snugly to protect the child properly.

Indoor Safety

One of the most important safety items in any area where children spend time is an emergency sticker on the phone. This sticker should include the telephone numbers of the police, fire department, ambulance, local hospital, physician, and poison control center in your area and your home address and telephone number.

Burns and Smoke Inhalation

Fires and burns are frequent causes of death and injury in children. The highest number of burn injuries occurs in the very young. Most burns are caused by a scald from a hot liquid. Many scalds occur in the kitchen when toddlers grab pot handles extending over the stove, spilling the boiling contents on themselves. Burns may also be inflicted (child abuse).

Children can also be scalded by hot water in sinks or tubs when a parent or caregiver leaves them alone momentarily or when another child bathes a younger child with water that is too hot. To prevent these injuries, reduce the temperature of your hot water heater to between 120°F and 130°F. (Most water heaters are pre-set at 150°F.) At 140°F, water takes only 6 seconds to cause a scald burn, whereas at 120°F, it takes 5 minutes to cause a scald burn.

Flame burns most commonly occur when a house catches fire or when bed sheets or clothing are ignited by open flames or ciga-rettes. Many burn injuries have been prevented with the develop-ment of flame-retardant children's sleepwear. Electric short circuits also may cause house fires and deaths. Do not use appliances with frayed cords or damaged plugs.

Most deaths and serious injuries in house fires are caused by smoke inhalation, which can be prevented by installing and main-taining smoke detectors on each level of the home or day-care center. Smoke detectors must have batteries, however, and these batteries must be changed twice every year. Develop a schedule to be sure your smoke detector batteries are changed. For example, change them every fall and spring when changing the clocks from and to daylight savings time.

Burns can also occur when a child comes into contact with hot irons, curling irons, or heating sources, such as woodstoves. These burns are preventable by keeping irons out of the child's reach and by placing a barrier around all woodstoves, hot radiators, and other heating sources.

Falls

Falls are the most frequent cause of injury to children younger than 6 years. About 200 children die from falls each year.

A common fall occurs when a baby climbs out of a crib. Many crib injuries, in fact, result from an unsafe crib. A small child can sustain a fracture if arm, leg, or head becomes wedged between the crib rails and the mattress. In some such cases the child can suffocate. Infants can die from strangulation if their heads become caught between the widely spaced bars of some older cribs or if clothing becomes caught on finials (corner posts) that extend above the side rail.

Twenty percent of all falls occur on stairs. It is important to keep stairways as safe as possible by providing adequate lighting, removing toys, tacking down loose carpet, and using appropriate gate enclosures. Avoid the accordion-type gate with wide gaps at the top. Instead, use a safety gate that is permanently mounted or firmly attached to the wall with double closures that cannot be operated by children. Use of infant walkers is discouraged because of the dangers they create, especially near stairs or ramps.

Children may also suffer permanent injury and death by falling from upper-floor windows. Open such windows only from the top or 4 to 5 inches up from the bottom and secure them at the proper height with a burglar lock available at any hardware store. Gates should be placed over the lower portion of windows in high-rise buildings.

Firearms

Injuries from firearms are a leading cause of death and permanent injury in children and adolescents, and these injuries have been increasing at an alarming rate. Most firearm injuries result from handguns, which can often be found in the home loaded and readily accessible to children (eg, under a pillow or in a drawer). An increasing number of injuries and deaths occur when children and adolescents take guns to school.

If a gun is kept in the home, adults should ensure that it cannot be found or operated by children. Homes of preadolescents and adolescents (10 years old or older) or persons with a history of violent behavior, depression, or drug or alcohol abuse are high-risk homes. Guns should be kept with increased caution and surveillance or not kept in these homes, because there is an increased likelihood that the gun will be associated with intentional or unintentional injury, homicide, or suicide.

When a gun is kept in any home it should be stored unloaded, and the ammunition should be stored in a location separate from the gun. Trigger locks or lockboxes should secure every gun in the home. The guns should be checked daily by an adult to ensure that children have not touched them, played with them, or taken them to school.

Poisoning

Childhood poisoning is a common problem in our society. We have access to more than 250 000 household products, many with harmful chemicals. Many of us have miniature drugstores in our homes and even in our desk drawers at work. It is not surprising that curious and exploring children are often victims of poisoning.

Some common poisons found in the home include

- Prescription and nonprescription medications, most importantly iron pills, vitamins containing iron, Tylenol, and aspirin
- Plants
- Cleansers, polishing agents, ammonia, and detergents
- Cosmetics and hair care products (ie, hair coloring agents)
- Alcohol and liquor
- Insect and rodent poisons, moth balls
- Gasoline, kerosene, and other petroleum products
- Pesticides, weed killers, and fertilizers
- Lye and acids
- Paint and paint thinners

The best place to obtain poison information is your regional poison control center. The staff there can provide accurate, up-to-date, and immediate information about almost any poisonous or potentially poisonous product. They will also provide immediate first-aid instructions and treatment recommendations. This service is available 24 hours a day. *You should be familiar with the telephone number of the poison control center in your area and post it near your telephone.*

Syrup of ipecac (to cause vomiting) should be kept in every home with young children. It is a helpful treatment for various types of poisoning, but it should be used *only when prescribed by a doctor or poison control center.* The vomiting can help the poisoned child and eliminate unnecessary and costly trips to an emergency facility. For some poison ingestions, inducing vomiting is *not* indicated and may be harmful. Always check with the poison control center or your doctor *before* giving ipecac.

Safe storage of medicine, vitamins, and household cleaning supplies is one of the most important methods of poison prevention. Poisons should *never* be stored in empty food or drink containers (eg, kerosene in cola bottles). These items should be stored in specially designed and labeled containers, in high places out of a child's sight and reach. Even high shelves that are thought to be safe have been reached by resourceful children who stack objects and climb to reach them. A high, locked cabinet is the best place to store poisons.

Many poison control centers report that their most frequent type of call involves children who have eaten plants. Eating or merely chewing on certain household plants can result in serious poisoning. Parents and caregivers should learn the names and toxicity of the plants in and around the home or childcare area and remove those that are poisonous.* Consult your local poison control center to determine if a plant (including stems, leaves, bulbs, flowers, fruit, nuts, seeds, and berries) is poisonous.

Toy Injuries

Most toy-related injuries occur from children falling on, tripping over, or being hit by toys. Choking from inhalation of small toys or parts of toys is the second most common toy injury. Half of the deaths from toy-related injuries involve children who choke on balloons, ride tricycles into pools, or are struck by motor vehicles while riding tricycles.

Electric or battery-powered toys can overheat, melt, and start fires, causing other toy-related injuries. Button-shaped batteries (eg, for watches or cameras) will often cause severe tissue damage if ingested and can burn tissue if placed in body cavities. Call your poison control center if such a battery is swallowed or becomes lodged in a child's body.

Choking and Suffocation

Choking and suffocation are among the most common causes of preventable death in children younger than 1 year and a common cause of death in children younger than 14 years.

Choking is caused by the inhalation of food or objects. Strangulation or suffocation is caused by constriction about the neck or blockage of the nose, mouth, or windpipe (trachea). Choking, strangulation, or suffocation results in blockage of the airway passages, which interferes with breathing. This can cause death or brain damage.

---

*See Ogzewalla CD, Bonfiglio JF, Sigell LT. Common plants and their toxicity. *Pediatr Clin North Am.* 1987;34:1557-1598.

The most common objects that choke, strangle, or suffocate children are

- Food items, such as hot dogs, grapes, nuts, popcorn, and hard candy. Formula, milk, or juice can cause choking if these liquids are given to an infant who is lying down, especially from a propped bottle.
- Toys and parts of toys that are small enough to place in the mouth. Uninflated balloons or pieces of balloons are frequent causes of choking and can be particularly hard to remove.
- A variety of other small items, such as coins, marbles, buttons, beads, safety pins
- Drapery and extension cords
- Plastic bags
- Cords from which toys and objects such as rattles, pacifiers, and jewelry are hung around the child's neck

Drowning

Drowning is a major cause of accidental death in children. Drowning is suffocation by immersion in water, resulting in death. The household bath is the most common site for drowning in the first year of life. Infants, toddlers, and preschoolers must always be supervised by an adult in the bath or near any container of water, including buckets and toilets. They should not be left alone near the water. Toilet lids should be closed, and industrial buckets (5 gallons or more) should be made inaccessible to toddlers. Young children can drown in only a few inches of water.

Outdoor Safety

When children play outdoors, they are expected to be active. We can help prevent injuries by following some simple safety guidelines.

Most important, children should play away from streets. This eliminates the temptation to follow a ball or other toy into the street. Toddlers playing outside should always be supervised, and young children playing near animals must always be with an adult.

Drownings

Drownings in backyard swimming pools are a leading cause of death and permanent brain damage in children, particularly among infants and toddlers. A toddler is by nature inquisitive, and water offers exciting possibilities. The natural curiosity of toddlers, their inability to appreciate the danger and depth of water, and the attraction of water play can be a dangerous combination. The young child is capable of getting into a swimming pool alone but may be incapable of getting out and may become helpless in the water.

Access to swimming pools should be carefully controlled. All pools, hot tubs, and spas should be surrounded by a nonclimbable fence at least 5 feet high, with a self-closing, self-latching gate. You *must not* consider the house to be part of the fence, because toddlers may leave the house and find themselves in the pool area. Pool covers and pool alarms may give a false sense of security because they will not prevent drownings. Contrary to popular belief, the drowning child often sinks quietly without screaming for help. *Children should always be supervised when they play in or around water,* and all toys should be removed from the pool area at the end of every supervised swim period so that children are not lured back into the water. Parents and older children in a home with a swimming pool should learn CPR.

While on docks or at beaches or rivers, children should wear life vests. Children can fall into these waters suddenly and quietly. Children swimming in moving water should wear approved flotation devices. No child should ever swim alone.

Playground Injuries

The playground is a frequent site of childhood injury. The number and severity of these injuries can be reduced if we ensure that all playground equipment is safe. Attachments, cables, and seats of swings should be inspected regularly, particularly at the beginning and middle of every summer, and kept in good repair. Playgrounds should be built on energy-absorbing surfaces, such as sand, wood chips, or rubber padding. Concrete and grass *do not* provide adequate cushioning for children when they fall.

Safety Checklist

The checklist in Appendix B has been developed to help you make a child's daily environment as safe as possible. It is based on the most up-to-date injury information available and is designed to guide you through an inspection of your home, day-care center, school, baby-sitter's home, or wherever a child spends time. Take it with you on your inspection tour and circle the appropriate answers to the questions. You may be surprised to detect several potential dangers that you can remedy.

Conclusions

This safety section is intended to alert you to some of the hazards in your child's environment. You can help prevent injury and death to the children around you by following the recommendations of your course instructor and those listed in the checklist.

The following safety supplies are recommended for any area where children spend time:

- Syrup of ipecac to use in certain types of poisoning
- Plastic plug covers for electric outlets to protect children from electric shock
- Plastic outlet covers to use when an electric cord is plugged into the outlet
- Cabinet latches and locks to keep children away from medicines, cleaning supplies, knives, etc
- Emergency telephone numbers for quick dialing in case of an emergency
- A smoke detector with working battery to provide early warning and help reduce fire deaths
- A hot-water gauge (such as a meat or candy thermometer) for measuring the temperature of tap water to prevent scalding
- An out-of-reach hook-and-eye latch to prevent children from gaining entry to the basement or garage, where dangerous products are often stored

These safety devices will not only help reduce childhood injuries, but they will also give you the immediate satisfaction of knowing that you have taken steps to improve the safety of a child's environment.

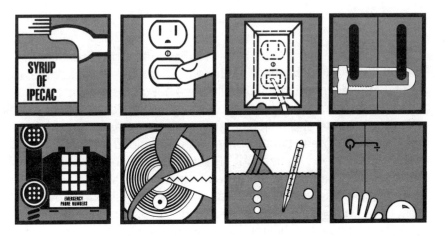

3
Prudent Heart Living: You Are in Control

Heart disease is the No. 1 killer of Americans. This disease is thought to begin in childhood and progress through adolescence and young adulthood, but it usually does not cause any visible symptoms until middle adulthood. Even young children, however, may demonstrate or develop conditions that increase the risk of heart disease. These conditions include high blood pressure and high levels of blood cholesterol. "Prudent heart living" is a lifestyle designed to minimize the risk of future heart disease.

Many risks associated with heart disease are influenced by lifestyle — what you eat, how much you exercise, and how you care for your health. Children begin developing lifestyle patterns at an early age. Once developed, the patterns are difficult to change. You can't begin preventing heart disease too soon.

Children often choose to eat junk food and other high-fat foods, unless they are taught the importance of eating nutritious food. With such an understanding and many opportunities to practice positive eating habits, children will be able to make wise choices and encourage others to do the same. Children should be taught at an early age the importance of a healthy diet, regular exercise, and regular medical care.

Children learn from the attitudes, behavior, and lifestyles of the adults around them. You are a model for them. The best way to encourage positive attitudes and behavior about food, physical activity, and rest is to practice what you preach. As you model positive health habits and encourage these habits in children, you will reduce your likelihood of heart disease also.

Important risk factors for heart disease are smoking, a diet rich in saturated fats and cholesterol, sedentary living, and high blood pressure.

Smoking

Exposure to tobacco smoke is the most preventable cause of heart and lung disease in the United States. The risk of heart disease is directly related to the number of cigarettes a person smokes daily and the amount of exposure to the smoking of others. People who smoke a pack of cigarettes a day have more than twice the risk of heart disease as a person who has never smoked. The risk is even greater in people who also have high blood pressure and high levels of cholesterol in their blood. Tobacco smoke is also harmful to nonsmokers in the household. Second-hand smoke ("passive smoking") can actually cause infants to develop respiratory problems and can worsen asthma and other respiratory diseases in children and adults.

Children develop attitudes about smoking at an early age and imitate the behavior of their parents or primary caregivers. Research shows that children of parents who smoke are more likely to smoke than children of nonsmokers.

If you smoke, try to stop completely or reduce the number of cigarettes you smoke daily. If you quit smoking, it will reduce your risk of heart disease, eliminate the effects of passive smoking on other members of the household, and set a good example of healthy behavior for your children. While you are trying to quit smoking, smoke only outside or in well-ventilated areas, and don't smoke in the car. This is important for the health of your children and anyone in the home with respiratory disease. Tobacco smoke accumulates in household furnishings (including draperies, upholstery, and carpeting) and may take as long as 3 to 6 months to disappear, so the effects of passive smoking on your family may not disappear immediately after you quit smoking.

Diet

Children begin to develop lifelong eating habits and attitudes toward food at an early age. Eating habits established during childhood are hard to change. They affect two major risk factors associated with heart disease: high blood cholesterol and high blood pressure. Diets high in cholesterol and saturated fats contribute to high blood cholesterol levels. Obesity and excessive salt intake contribute to high blood pressure.

Because diet is a major risk factor in the development of heart disease, the AHA is especially concerned with helping children develop positive attitudes about nutritious foods.

The AHA recommends that you consume foods low in cholesterol and saturated fats, eat a variety of foods every day, prevent obesity by limiting calorie intake to the amount needed for normal growth and development, limit salt intake, and reduce the amount of fat in the diet.

To reduce the amount of fat in the diet:

- Limit meat, seafood, and poultry to 6 ounces per day.
- Use skinless chicken, turkey, or fish in most main dishes.
- Choose lean cuts of meat and remove visible fat.
- Substitute meatless or low-meat main dishes for regular entrees.
- Use no more than 5 to 8 teaspoons of oil or fat per day.
- Use skim milk and low-fat cheese.

To help control cholesterol:

- Eat no more than three egg yolks per week.
- Limit use of shrimp, lobster, and organ meats (ie, liver, heart).

When you reduce the amount of saturated fat in your diet, a higher percentage of total calories must come from other sources — proteins and carbohydrates. If carbohydrates provide the extra calories, complex carbohydrates (cereals, fruits, and vegetables) are recommended rather than sugar. Although sugar is not a risk factor for heart disease, it is associated with increased risk of tooth decay and obesity.

Children tend to like or dislike foods their parents like or dislike. To encourage good eating habits, set a good example by eating nutritious foods and trying new and different foods. Be casual about introducing a new food. Encourage children to taste it, but don't force the issue. To make vegetables appealing to children, try serving them raw. Cut them into interesting shapes and serve them with low-fat dips or sauces.

Avoid candy, chips, soft drinks, and other foods that are high in calories but low in nutrients. Offer apple wedges, bananas, carrots, and other fruits and vegetables for snacks. Encourage children to drink water and natural juices rather than soft drinks.

Limit the amount of fried food in the diet. Bake or broil meats. Use a variety of seasonings to create a variety of tastes. When you do fry food, use vegetable oil.

A calm, unhurried atmosphere at mealtime helps children develop positive attitudes toward food. Allow children to serve themselves, with help as needed. Provide small portions and let children ask for seconds. Avoid overwhelming children with servings that are too large. Don't encourage children to "clean" their plates because this can encourage overeating. Make sure children do not substitute snack foods high in fats or salt for meals.

Serve a variety of foods at meals, including fruit, vegetables, cereals, pasta, low-fat dairy products, fish, poultry, and lean meats.

Following these guidelines and reducing risk factors may reduce the risk of heart attack or stroke. At the very least, the result will be good general health and physical fitness for every member of the family. Children will benefit most by learning the habits of prudent heart living early in life.

The AHA publishes other materials that further explain the essentials of prudent heart living. Contact your local AHA affiliate for details.

Physical Activity

Children begin to control their bodies and use them effectively in the preschool years. By age 6 most children have mastered movements basic to developing sport skills in later childhood and adulthood. At the same time children are developing attitudes about physical activity and its importance in daily life. Children who enjoy movement and physical activity usually continue to enjoy them into adulthood. Also, children who know that physical activity is important to health probably will include it as a regular part of their adult lives.

A regular program of aerobic physical activity strengthens the heart so that it pumps more blood per beat. This allows the heart to beat at a slower rate.

Physical activity improves blood circulation throughout the body so that the heart, lungs, and other organs work together more effectively. Physical activity is also important in controlling weight and reducing stress.

Some children are naturally active, given opportunity and encouragement. Such children probably do not require a structured exercise program for cardiovascular fitness. However, they do need opportunities to walk, run, jump, kick, throw, and catch. Activities should correspond to each child's abilities and interests and should be fun. As children engage in physical activity, they will begin to understand how such movement helps them become stronger and healthier.

Adults should set a good example for children by exercising regularly. Climb stairs instead of taking the elevator. If you must go up or down several flights, climb two or three and then take the elevator. Walk short distances to the store and other places instead of driving. You and your child will benefit from such activities.

Rest is also important for healthy heart living. Encourage quiet activities such as reading and working puzzles. Adequate sleep is equally important to health.

High Blood Pressure

High blood pressure is directly related to the development of heart disease. When high blood pressure is combined with other risk factors, such as obesity or exposure to tobacco smoke, the risk of heart attack or stroke is greatly increased.

If you have not had your blood pressure checked recently, now is the time to do it. Children, adolescents, and adults should have their blood pressure checked as part of their regular medical check-ups. High blood pressure can be controlled, and there is evidence that control of high blood pressure will reduce the risk of heart disease.

4
Normal Heart and Lung Anatomy and Function

The heart, a muscle about the size of a clenched fist, is located in the center of the chest behind the breastbone (sternum) and in front of the spine. It has four chambers with valves that regulate the flow of blood through the heart chambers and into the pulmonary artery and the aorta. The aorta and other arteries carry blood away from the heart and connect to small blood vessels called *capillaries* in the body organs. The capillaries join together to form veins that carry blood back to the heart and into the lungs by way of the pulmonary artery. The coronary arteries are special arteries that supply blood to the heart muscle itself.

Location of the Heart

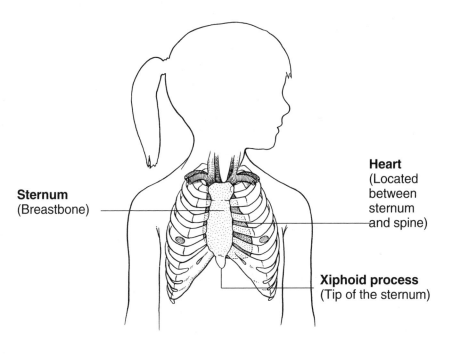

Sternum
(Breastbone)

Heart
(Located between sternum and spine)

Xiphoid process
(Tip of the sternum)

The Heart and Circulatory System

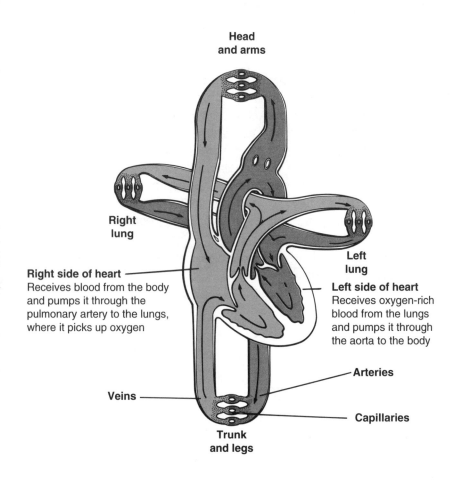

Head and arms

Right lung

Right side of heart
Receives blood from the body and pumps it through the pulmonary artery to the lungs, where it picks up oxygen

Left lung

Left side of heart
Receives oxygen-rich blood from the lungs and pumps it through the aorta to the body

Arteries

Veins

Capillaries

Trunk and legs

The function of the heart is to pump blood to the lungs, where it picks up oxygen, and to pump the oxygen-enriched blood to all parts of the body. The heart pumps approximately 5 quarts (almost equal to 5 liters) of blood per minute in an adult. All cells of the body require oxygen to carry out their normal functions. When the heart stops (cardiac arrest), oxygen is not circulated, and the oxygen stored in the brain and other vital organs is used up quickly.

The heartbeat is triggered by natural electric impulses sent through the heart 60 to 150 times a minute. The younger the child, the more rapid the heartbeat. During exercise the heart of the average adult can pump up to 25½ quarts (about 25 liters) each minute. Less blood is pumped by the heart of a physically active child, but the amount of blood pumped is proportionate to size.

The lungs are basically air sacs (alveoli) surrounded by capillaries. Nerve impulses from the brain to the chest muscles and the diaphragm cause breathing. With each breath air is carried through the airways (nose, mouth, throat, larynx, trachea, and bronchi) and into the air sacs of the lungs.

Parts of the Airway

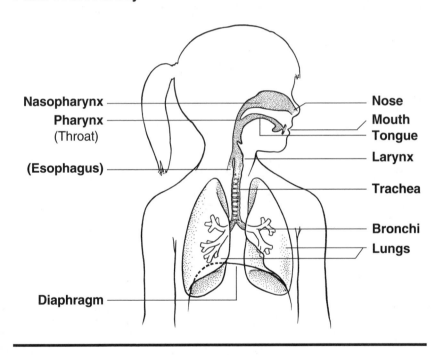

Air at sea level is approximately 21% oxygen. As breathing fills the air sacs, the blood around the air sacs picks up the oxygen and carries it back to the heart, which pumps it throughout the body. As oxygen is taken from the blood by cells in the body, carbon dioxide is given off as a waste product. Carbon dioxide is returned by the blood to the air sacs and exhaled out of the body. Normally, the blood picks up only one fourth of the oxygen in the air. The rest is exhaled. This is why mouth-to-mouth breathing can provide the victim with enough oxygen (about 16% oxygen) to help support life.

When breathing stops (respiratory arrest), the heart may continue to pump blood for several minutes, carrying existing stores of oxygen to the brain and the rest of the body. Early, prompt rescue efforts for the victim of respiratory arrest or choking (foreign-body airway obstruction) can prevent the heart from stopping (cardiac arrest) and maintain oxygen delivery to the brain and body.

5
Introduction to CPR Techniques

CPR involves a combination of mouth-to-mouth rescue breathing (or other artificial ventilation techniques) and chest compressions to help the victim of sudden respiratory or cardiac arrest survive until advanced life support care can be provided. CPR keeps some oxygenated blood flowing to the brain and other vital organs until medical treatment can restore normal heart action.

Heart disease is rare in infants and children and an uncommon cause of cardiac arrest in children. Instead, the typical cause of cardiac arrest in infants and children is lack of oxygen supply to the heart muscle caused by a breathing problem, respiratory arrest, or shock. Breathing problems can occur because of choking, suffocation, airway disease, lung disease, near-drowning, or injuries involving the airway or brain. If a child stops breathing, cardiac arrest follows in a very short time. If breathing assistance is provided for such a victim, cardiac arrest may actually be prevented.

If CPR is started promptly and advanced life support is available quickly, the victim has a chance to survive. CPR includes three basic rescue skills, known as the ABCs of CPR: Airway, Breathing, and Circulation.

Airway

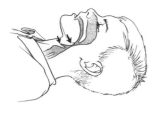

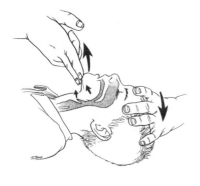

When a person loses consciousness, the muscles relax and the tongue falls backward and obstructs the airway. Therefore, the first action for successful resuscitation is to open the airway. It is important to remember that the back of the tongue and other structures in the back of the throat are the most common cause of airway obstruction in the unconscious victim. Since these structures are all attached to the lower jaw, the airway can usually be opened by tilting the victim's head back and moving the lower jaw (chin) up and outward. This action lifts the tongue and its attachments from the back of the throat.

Breathing

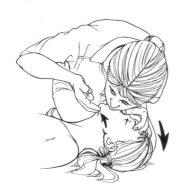

When breathing stops, only a small amount of oxygen remains in the lungs and bloodstream. Therefore, when breathing stops, cardiac arrest and death quickly follow. Mouth-to-mouth rescue breathing is the quickest way to get oxygen into the victim's lungs. The air you breathe into the victim contains enough oxygen to supply the victim's needs. Rescue breathing must be performed until the victim can breathe on his or her own or until trained professionals take over. *Remember:* If the victim's heart is beating, you must (1) maintain an open airway and (2) breathe at a rate of once every 3 seconds for infants or children (20 times per minute). If the victim's heart is not beating, you will have to perform mouth-to-mouth rescue breathing *plus* chest compressions.

Circulation

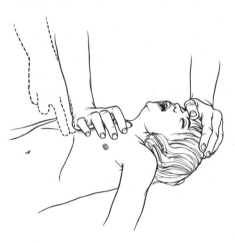

The third skill of CPR is chest compressions, which help to circulate blood and maintain some blood flow to the lungs, brain, heart, and other vital organs. Whenever chest compressions are performed, mouth-to-mouth rescue breathing or rescue breathing provided with medical equipment by EMS personnel must also be performed.

6

Relief of Foreign-Body Airway Obstruction

Airway obstruction (choking) remains a common cause of death and disability in children. A complete airway obstruction means that the breathing passages are totally blocked and the victim is unable to speak, cough, or breathe. It is important to recognize signs of distress and respond quickly and effectively. You will learn how to give first aid to victims of choking. These procedures are different for infant and child victims. The maneuvers for both are described in chapter 7.

Causes

A variety of foods and foreign bodies can obstruct a child's airway. The most common causes of airway obstruction are toys, small parts of toys, balloons, and foods such as hot dogs, round candies, nuts, and grapes. Airway obstruction may also occur when illnesses such as epiglottitis or croup cause the air passages to swell and narrow, but these diseases require medical attention and will not be relieved by the techniques you are about to learn.

Prevention

Many incidents of choking in children can be prevented by following these guidelines:

- Prevent children from walking, running, playing, or crying with food or foreign objects in their mouths.
- Keep small objects (marbles, beads, small toys, thumbtacks, etc) away from infants and preschool children.
- Serve each infant and child food that is appropriate for his or her age and size. Avoid nuts, popcorn, and small, hard candies before age 4.
- Cut children's food into small pieces.
- Teach children to chew slowly and thoroughly and to not laugh and talk while eating.

Recognition of Foreign-Body Airway Obstruction

Airway obstruction should be suspected in an infant or child who *suddenly* chokes and begins to cough, gag, or have high-pitched noisy breathing. An older child may also use the "universal distress signal" of choking: clutching the neck between the thumb and index finger. You may ask the child if he or she is choking, and the child may nod.

Airway obstruction may be partial or complete. In *partial* airway obstruction, air exchange may be good or poor. The child may be able to cough, although there may be wheezing between coughs. *If a child is coughing vigorously, the airway is only partially obstructed. Do not attempt to relieve the obstruction.* As long as air exchange continues to be good, do not interfere, but take the child to a physician or medical center.

Poor air exchange is characterized by an ineffective cough, high-pitched noises while inhaling, increasing breathing difficulty, and blueness of the lips, nails, and skin. When these signs are observed, treat the infant or child as though he or she has a complete airway obstruction.

If the infant or child has a *complete* airway obstruction, no air can be expelled, so he or she will be *unable to make a sound. The infant or child with complete airway obstruction requires immediate help to relieve the obstruction.*

Maneuvers

The maneuvers described on pages 50-59 should be performed when an infant or child demonstrates *complete* airway obstruction and aspiration of a foreign body is witnessed or strongly suspected (eg, after attempts to ventilate fail). The infant or child may be conscious or may lose consciousness as you begin to help.

The maneuvers are also appropriate when an unconscious, non-breathing child is found and the airway remains obstructed despite attempts to open it.

Not all airway obstruction is caused by a foreign object. Infections may cause airway swelling and obstruction that will not be relieved by the maneuvers described here. Children with an *infectious* cause of airway obstruction need prompt medical attention in a hospital's emergency department, and time should not be wasted on a futile attempt to relieve the obstruction.

7

The Performance Guidelines and How to Use Them

This section provides performance guidelines. These are designed to help you learn the basic emergency procedures taught in this course. If your course teaches maneuvers for both infants and children, you will need to study all the performance guidelines. If you are taking a course that emphasizes maneuvers for an infant *or* a child, you will need to study only those performance guidelines that relate to the information presented in your course. If you have any questions about which guidelines to study, ask your instructor for help.

The performance guidelines will give you the specific steps necessary to do the following:

- Perform CPR on an infant whose breathing or pulse has stopped (pages 32-39)
- Perform CPR on a child whose breathing or pulse has stopped (pages 40-49)
- Clear an infant's airway if it is obstructed by foreign material (pages 50-69)
- Clear a child's airway if it is obstructed by foreign material (pages 70-85)

This section contains pictures of each important step as well as a description of the step, guidelines for performance, and the reason for the step. Use this section

- *Before* you take a CPR course to help you prepare for what is ahead
- *During* your CPR course as you practice with a manikin
- *After* you have finished the course to refresh your memory

CPR, like any skill, should be practiced occasionally to keep the important steps straight. Then if an emergency arises, you may be able to help save a life. Refresh your skills at least every 1 to 2 years by contacting an AHA office and taking a refresher course.

It will take only a little of your time, and you will feel good knowing that you are still able to perform CPR. A refresher course also keeps you informed about advances in CPR technique.

Never rehearse or practice CPR on another person!

Reading material does not, by itself, constitute a CPR course. It is necessary to practice with manikins, with trained instructors to guide you, to gain the skills of CPR.

Performance Guidelines

	Objectives
	Assessment: Determine unresponsiveness. Shout for help.
	Action: Position the infant on his or her back.
	Action: Open the airway (head tilt–chin lift). **Assessment:** Determine breathlessness.

Critical Performance	Reason
Tap or gently shake victim's shoulder. Call out "Help!" If help arrives, send someone to activate the EMS system.	You do not want to begin CPR unnecessarily if the infant is sleeping. A call for help will summon persons nearby but allow you to begin CPR if necessary.
Turn the infant as a unit, supporting head and neck. Place the infant on a firm surface. If the infant's head or neck has possibly been injured, turn the infant carefully, holding the head and neck as a unit to avoid bending or turning the neck.	For CPR to be effective, the infant must be flat on his or her back on a firm surface. CPR cannot be performed if the infant is face down.
Lift the chin up and out gently with one hand while pushing down on the forehead with the other to tilt the head back into a neutral position. Don't close the mouth. If trauma is suspected, use the jaw thrust to open the airway.	The airway must be opened to determine whether the infant is breathing. Infants may be unable to breathe because the tongue is obstructing the airway.
Maintain an open airway. Turn your head toward the infant's chest with your ear directly over and close to the infant's mouth. *Look* at the chest for movement. *Listen* for the sounds of breathing. *Feel* for breath on your cheek.	Hearing and feeling are the only true ways of determining the presence of effective breathing. If there is chest movement but you cannot feel or hear air, the airway may still be obstructed. Rescue breathing should not be performed on someone who is breathing effectively.

Performance Guidelines

Objectives

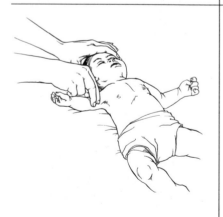

Action: If the victim is not breathing, provide rescue breathing. Give 2 slow rescue breaths (1 to 1½ seconds per breath). Observe the rise of the chest with each breath.

Assessment: Determine pulselessness.

Critical Performance	Reason
Maintain pressure on the infant's forehead to keep the head tilted. With the other hand lift the chin, open your mouth wide and take a deep breath. Cover the infant's mouth and nose with your mouth, making a tight seal. Breathe into the infant's mouth and nose twice, completely refilling your lungs between breaths. Watch for the infant's chest to rise. Each rescue breath is given over 1 to 1½ seconds, allowing the infant's lungs to deflate between breaths. If the rescue breaths do not cause the infant's chest to rise, the airway is obstructed. Reposition the head, lift the chin, and try again. If the chest still does not rise with the rescue breath, start the relief of obstructed airway sequence (page 50).	It is important to get as much oxygen as possible into the infant. If your rescue breathing is effective, you will • Feel air going in as you blow • Feel the air leaving your own lungs • See the infant's chest rise and fall The most common cause of an obstructed airway is that the airway has not been properly opened.
Place 2 or 3 fingers on the inside of the infant's upper arm, between the elbow and shoulder. Press gently on the inside of the arm with your index and middle fingers. Maintain head tilt with the other hand. Feel for the brachial pulse. • If pulse is present and breathing has not resumed, breathe for the infant at the rate of 20 times per minute. • If there is no pulse, start chest compressions.	This step should not take more than a few seconds. If the heart is beating effectively, you should be able to feel a strong, rapid pulse within a few seconds. If you do not feel a pulse, begin chest compressions.

Performance Guidelines

	Objectives
	Action: Begin the first cycle of chest compressions.

Critical Performance	Reason
To begin the first cycle, imagine a line drawn between the infant's nipples. Place 2 or 3 fingers on the breastbone (sternum) about 1 finger's width below that line. Because of wide variations in the relative sizes of rescuers' hands and infants' chests, these instructions are only guidelines. After finding the position for compressions, make sure your fingers are not over the bottom of the sternum (xiphoid). Compress the infant's chest downward approximately one third to one half the depth of the chest (about ½ to 1 inch, but these measurements are not precise) at least 100 times per minute.	Proper finger placement is important to maximize the effectiveness of compressions and minimize the risk of injury to the infant.
Compress smoothly and evenly, and release pressure between compressions to allow the chest to return to its normal position. Do not lift your fingers off the chest.	With each compression, you want to squeeze the heart and increase pressure within the chest so that blood moves to the vital organs.
To achieve a proper rate and ratio, count aloud: "one-two-three-four-five-breathe . . . ."	

Performance Guidelines

	Objectives
	Action: Give **5** compressions and **1** breath.
	Action: Activate the EMS system at the end of 20 cycles or 20 rescue breaths (approximately 1 minute). After EMS notification, resume CPR, beginning with chest compressions. Check every few minutes for return of pulse.

Critical Performance	Reason
Ventilate properly. After every **5** compressions, deliver **1** rescue breath. Pause briefly after each 5th compression to deliver the 1 breath.	Adequate oxygenation must be maintained.
Know your local EMS telephone number. If a second person is available, he or she should telephone the local EMS immediately while you continue CPR. If you are alone, perform CPR for approximately 1 minute *before* activating the EMS system. • If the pulse returns, check for spontaneous breathing. — If there is no breathing, give 1 rescue breath every 3 seconds (20 breaths per minute) and monitor the pulse. — If breathing resumes, maintain an open airway and monitor breathing and pulse. • If pulse *and* breathing resume and are regular and there is no evidence of trauma, turn the infant on his or her side, continue to monitor breathing and pulse, and await rescue personnel.	Notification of the EMS system at this time allows the caller to give complete information about the infant's condition.

Performance Guidelines

CPR: Child (1 to 8 years)

	Objectives
	Assessment: Determine unresponsiveness. Shout for help.
	Action: Position the child on his or her back.
	Action: Open the airway (head tilt–chin lift). **Assessment:** Determine breathlessness.

Critical Performance	Reason
Tap or gently shake the shoulder. Shout "Are you OK?" Call out "Help!" If help arrives, send someone to activate the EMS system.	One concern is the risk of possible damage from unnecessary CPR for children who are sleeping. A call for help will summon people nearby but allow you to begin CPR if necessary.
Turn the child as a unit, supporting head and neck. If head or neck injury is suspected, do not bend or turn the neck.	For CPR to be effective, the child must be flat on his or her back on a firm, hard surface. CPR cannot be performed if the child is face down.
Kneel beside the child's shoulder. Lift the chin up gently with one hand while pushing down on the forehead with the other to tilt the head back into a neutral position. Do not close the mouth. If there is evidence of trauma, open the airway using a jaw thrust.	The airway must be opened to determine whether the child is breathing. Children may be unable to breathe because the tongue is obstructing the airway.
Maintain an open airway. Turn your head toward the child's chest with your ear directly over and close to the child's mouth. _Look_ at the chest for movement. _Listen_ for the sounds of breathing. _Feel_ for breath on your cheek.	Hearing and feeling are the only true ways of determining the presence of effective breathing. If there is chest movement but you cannot feel or hear air, the airway may still be obstructed. Rescue breathing should not be performed on someone who is breathing effectively.

Performance Guidelines

CPR: Child (1 to 8 years) (continued)

	Objectives
	Objectives **Action:** If the child is not breathing, provide rescue breathing. Give 2 rescue breaths (1 to 1½ seconds per breath). Observe the rise of the chest with each breath.

Critical Performance	Reason
Pinch the child's nostrils closed with the thumb and forefinger of the hand maintaining pressure on the child's forehead while lifting the chin with the other hand. Open your mouth wide, take a deep breath, and make a tight seal over the child's mouth. Breathe into the child's mouth twice, completely refilling your lungs between breaths. Watch for the child's chest to rise. Each rescue breath is given over 1 to 1½ seconds, allowing the child's lungs to deflate between breaths.	It is important to get as much oxygen as possible into the child. If your rescue breathing is effective, you will • Feel air going in as you blow • Feel the air leaving your own lungs • See the child's chest rise and fall
If the rescue breaths do not cause the child's chest to rise, the airway is obstructed. Reposition the head, lift the chin, and try again. If the chest still does not rise with the rescue breath, start the relief of obstructed airway sequence (page 70).	Improper head tilt–chin lift is the most common reason that airway obstruction is not relieved.

Objectives

Assessment: Determine pulselessness.

Critical Performance	Reason
Using the hand that is farther from the child's forehead, place 2 or 3 fingers on the child's Adam's apple (voice box) just below the chin. Slide the fingers into the groove between the Adam's apple and the neck muscle on the side of the neck near you. Maintain head tilt with the other hand. Feel for the carotid pulse. • If a pulse is present and breathing has not resumed, breathe for the child at a rate of 20 times per minute. • If there is no pulse, start chest compressions.	This step should not take more than a few seconds. If the heart is beating effectively, you should feel a strong, rapid pulse within a few seconds. If you do not feel a pulse, begin chest compressions.

Performance Guidelines

	Objectives
	Action: Begin the first cycle of chest compressions.

Critical Performance	Reason
To begin the first cycle: Move the hand that is not maintaining head tilt to the child's chest. Place the heel of the hand on the lower half of the breastbone (sternum). Do not place your hand over the very bottom of the sternum (the xiphoid). Compress the child's chest downward approximately one third to one half the depth of the chest (this is about 1 to 1½ inches, but these measurements are not precise) at a rate of 100 times per minute.	Proper hand placement is important to maximize effective compressions and minimize the risk of injury to the child.
Compress smoothly and evenly, keeping your fingers off the child's ribs. Between compressions, release pressure and allow the chest to return to its normal position, but do not lift the hand off the chest. Say a mnemonic to maintain the proper rate and ratio. Count aloud to establish a rhythm: "one-two-three-four-five-breathe . . . ."	With each compression, you want to squeeze the heart and increase pressure within the chest so that blood moves to the vital organs.

CPR: Child (1 to 8 years) (continued)

	Objectives
	Action: Give **5** compressions and **1** breath.
	Action: Activate the EMS system at the end of 20 cycles or 20 rescue breaths (approximately 1 minute of CPR). After EMS activation, resume CPR, beginning with chest compressions. Check every few minutes for return of pulse.

Critical Performance	Reason
Ventilate properly. After every **5** compressions, deliver **1** rescue breath.	Adequate oxygenation must be maintained.
Know your local EMS telephone number. If a second person is available, he or she should telephone the local EMS immediately.	Notification of the EMS system at this time allows the caller to give complete information about the child's condition.

• If the pulse returns, check for spontaneous breathing.
  — If there is no breathing, give 1 rescue breath every 3 seconds (20 breaths per minute) and monitor the pulse.
  — If breathing resumes, maintain an open airway and monitor breathing and pulse.
• If pulse *and* breathing resume and are regular and there is no evidence of trauma, turn the child to the side, continue to monitor breathing and pulse, and await emergency personnel.	

Performance Guidelines

Relief of Obstructed Airway: Conscious Infant
(younger than 1 year)

	Objectives
	Assessment: Determine *complete* airway obstruction either by observing sudden onset of signs of complete airway obstruction or by the circumstances in which the infant is found.
	If the infant is *unable* to cry or cough effectively: **Action:** Deliver up to 5 back blows.

Critical Performance	Reason
Rescuer must identify *complete* airway obstruction by the presence of breathing difficulty, an absent or ineffective cough, dusky color, and an inability to make sounds.	In the conscious infant it is essential to recognize the signs of *complete* airway obstruction and take prompt action.
If the infant is able to cough or cry, do not interfere with the infant's attempts to expel the object.	If the infant is able to cough or cry, air is getting through the trachea (windpipe) and the obstruction is *not* complete. In such a situation, you may make things worse by interfering.
Support the infant's head and neck with one hand firmly holding the jaw. Place the infant face down on your forearm, keeping the head lower than the trunk.	You must hold the infant's head firmly to avoid injury. The back blows increase pressure in the airway and may help dislodge the object.
With the heel of your free hand, deliver up to **5** back blows forcefully between the infant's shoulder blades.	

Performance Guidelines

	Objectives
	Action: Deliver up to 5 chest thrusts over the lower half of the sternum (avoid the xiphoid).
	Action: Repeat the sequence of 5 back blows and 5 chest thrusts until the object is expelled or until the infant becomes unconscious. Be persistent!

Critical Performance	Reason
Supporting the head, sandwich the infant between your hands and arms and turn the infant on his or her back, keeping the head lower than the trunk.	
Deliver up to **5** thrusts over the lower half of the breastbone, using the same landmarks as those for chest compression. Make sure your fingers are not placed over the very bottom of the sternum (xiphoid).	Such thrusts can force air upward into the airway from the lungs with enough pressure to expel the foreign object.
Deliver the chest thrusts more slowly than when doing chest compressions.	
Alternate these maneuvers in rapid sequence: • Back blows • Chest thrusts	Persistent attempts should be made to relieve the obstruction. As the infant becomes more deprived of oxygen, the airway muscles will relax, and maneuvers that were previously ineffective may become effective.

Performance Guidelines

Objectives

Assessment: Loss of consciousness in infant with complete airway obstruction. Shout for help.

Action: Perform tongue-jaw lift. Remove obstructing object if you see it.

Action: Attempt to give 2 rescue breaths. If unsuccessful, reposition the head and try again.

Action: Deliver up to 5 back blows.

Critical Performance	Reason
Call out "Help!" If someone comes, that person should activate the EMS system. Position infant on back.	This initial call will alert bystanders and may enable them to activate the EMS system while you try to relieve the obstruction.
Open the mouth using tongue-jaw lift by placing your thumb in the infant's mouth over the tongue. Lift the tongue and jaw outward. If you see a foreign body, remove it. *Do not* perform a blind finger sweep.	Remove the object if you see it. Blind finger sweeps should *not* be performed because they may push the obstructing object back into or further into the airway.
Open airway with head tilt–chin lift and try to give breaths. If the chest does not rise, reposition the head and try again to give rescue breaths.	You must ensure that the head is properly positioned before you decide that the airway is obstructed by a foreign body.
Deliver back blows with infant positioned face down (as before).	

Performance Guidelines

Relief of Obstructed Airway: Infant Becomes Unconscious (continued)

	Objectives
	Action: Deliver up to 5 chest thrusts over the lower half of the sternum (avoid the xiphoid).
	Action: Perform tongue-jaw lift. Remove object if seen.
	Action: After each series of 5 back blows and 5 chest thrusts, perform tongue-jaw lift and remove object if seen. Open the airway and try to give rescue breaths. If unsuccessful, reposition head and reattempt breaths.
	Action: Activate the EMS system after approximately 1 minute.

Critical Performance	Reason
Find finger position as for chest compressions and deliver up to 5 compressions.	
If you see the object, remove it. *Do not* perform blind finger sweeps.	Blind finger sweeps may push the object back into or further into the airway.
Repeat these steps until rescue breaths are given successfully. If you are alone, activate the EMS system after about 1 minute of efforts to clear the airway.	Some airway obstruction may be caused by incorrect head and neck position.
	Activation of the EMS system will ensure the arrival of trained personnel.

Performance Guidelines

Relief of Obstructed Airway: Infant Becomes Unconscious (continued)

	Objectives
	Action: When obstruction is removed, check for breathing and pulse.

Critical Performance	Reason

Open the airway and check for breathing.
 	
• If there is no breathing, give 2 breaths. Check for a pulse.
  — If a pulse is present, provide 20 breaths per minute and continue to monitor pulse.
  — If there is no pulse, begin cycles of compressions and breaths.
• If breathing resumes and there is no evidence of trauma, place the infant on one side in the recovery position and await the arrival of emergency personnel.	

Performance Guidelines

Relief of Obstructed Airway: Unconscious Infant
(younger than 1 year)

	Objectives
	Assessment: Determine unresponsiveness. Shout for help.
	Action: Position the infant on back.
	Action: Open the airway.
	Assessment: Determine breathlessness.

Critical Performance	Reason
Tap or gently shake the shoulder. Call out "Help!" If someone comes, send that person to activate the EMS system.	This initial call for help is to alert bystanders.
Turn on back as a unit, supporting head and neck.	
Use head tilt–chin lift maneuver to position the infant's head in a neutral position and open the airway.	
Place an ear over the infant's mouth and observe the chest. *Look* at the chest for movement. *Listen* for the sounds of breathing. *Feel* for breath on your cheek.	You must determine that the infant is not breathing.

Performance Guidelines

	Objectives
	Action: Try to give 2 rescue breaths. Observe the rise of the chest with each breath.
	Action: If rescue breaths are unsuccessful, try again.
	Action: Deliver up to 5 back blows.

Critical Performance	Reason
With your mouth, make a tight seal over the infant's mouth and nose. Attempt rescue breaths.	Complete airway obstruction by a foreign body is assumed if the infant with signs of airway obstruction becomes unconscious, but when the infant is found unconscious, an attempt must be made to get some air into the lungs. If the chest rises, the airway is open. If the chest does not rise, attempt to reposition the head.
Reposition the head and perform chin lift. Seal the mouth and nose properly and try again to give rescue breaths.	Improper head tilt–chin lift is the most common reason that airway obstruction is not relieved.
Position the infant and deliver up to 5 back blows.	You must hold the head firmly to avoid injury. The back blows increase pressure in the airway and may help dislodge the object.

Performance Guidelines

	Objectives
	Action: Deliver up to 5 chest thrusts over the lower half of the sternum (avoid the xiphoid).
	Action: Perform tongue-jaw lift. Check for a foreign object and remove it if you see it.

Critical Performance	Reason
Turn the victim onto his or her back. Find finger position as for chest compressions, and deliver up to 5 chest thrusts.	Such thrusts can force air upward into the airway from the lungs with enough pressure to expel the foreign body.
Open the mouth with a tongue-jaw lift by putting your thumb in the infant's mouth over the tongue. Lift the tongue and jaw forward with fingers wrapped around the lower jaw. If you see a foreign body, remove it. *Do not* perform blind finger sweeps.	A dislodged foreign body may now be manually accessible if it has not been expelled. Blind finger sweeps should not be performed because they may push the obstructing object back into or further into the airway.

Performance Guidelines

	## Objectives
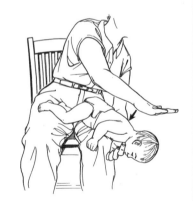	**Action:** Open airway and try to give rescue breaths. Repeat the sequence until successful or until emergency medical help arrives. Be persistent! If you are alone, activate the EMS system after approximately 1 minute of effort.

Critical Performance	Reason
Seal the mouth and nose properly and give rescue breaths.	By this time another attempt must be made to get some air into the lungs.
If the airway remains obstructed, alternate the following maneuvers in rapid sequence: • Deliver back blows. • Deliver chest thrusts. • Perform tongue-jaw lift, check for foreign body, and remove it if seen. • Open the airway. • Attempt, reattempt rescue breathing while maintaining an open airway.	You must try again to dislodge the foreign body and give rescue breaths. Persistent attempts should be made in sequence to relieve the obstruction. As the infant becomes more deprived of oxygen, the muscles will relax, and maneuvers that were previously ineffective may become effective.
Alternative Method for Infant Obstructed Airway Maneuver If your hands are small, you may find it physically difficult to perform the back blows and chest thrusts in the described manner, especially if the infant is large. An alternative method is to lay the infant face down on your lap, with the head lower than the trunk, making sure the head is firmly supported. After you have delivered the back blows, turn the infant face up and perform the chest thrusts.	

Performance Guidelines

	Objectives
	Action: When obstruction is removed, check for breathing and pulse.

Critical Performance	Reason
Open the airway and check for breathing. • If there is no breathing, give 2 breaths. Check for a pulse. — If a pulse is present, provide 20 breaths per minute and continue to monitor pulse. — If there is no pulse, begin cycles of compressions and breaths. • If breathing resumes and there is no evidence of trauma, place the infant on one side in the recovery position and await the arrival of emergency personnel.	

Performance Guidelines

Relief of Obstructed Airway: Conscious Child (1 to 8 years)

	Objectives
	Assessment: Determine *complete* airway obstruction by observing sudden onset of signs, including ineffective cough, increasing breathing difficulty, or blueness of lips, nails, or skin.
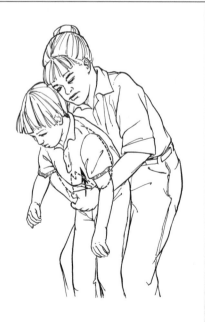	**Action:** If a cough is absent or ineffective: perform the Heimlich maneuver until the foreign body is expelled or the child becomes unconscious. Be persistent!

Critical Performance	Reason
The child is unable to speak or cough effectively. The rescuer asks "Are you choking?" The child may be using the universal distress signal of choking: clutching the neck between the thumb and index finger. *If the child is able to speak or cough effectively, do not interfere* with his or her attempts to expel the object.	In the conscious child, it is essential to recognize the signs of complete airway obstruction and take prompt action. If the child is able to speak or cough, air is getting past the obstruction and the obstruction is not complete. In such a situation you may make things worse by interfering.
The Heimlich maneuver: Stand behind the child and wrap your arms around the child's waist. Grasp one fist with your other hand and place the thumb side of your fist in the child's midline slightly above the navel but below the xiphoid and ribs. Press your fist into the child's abdomen with quick inward and upward thrusts. Each abdominal thrust should be delivered decisively, with the intent of relieving the obstruction. Several thrusts may be necessary to expel the object.	Such thrusts can force air upward from the lungs into the airway with enough pressure to expel the foreign body. Persistent attempts should be made in sequence to relieve the obstruction. As the child becomes more deprived of oxygen, the muscles will relax, and maneuvers that were previously ineffective may become effective.

Performance Guidelines

	## Objectives
	Assessment: Loss of consciousness in child with complete airway obstruction.
	Action: Place victim on back. Perform tongue-jaw lift. Remove foreign body if you see it.
	Action: Open airway and try to give 2 rescue breaths. If unsuccessful, reposition the head and try again.

Critical Performance	Reason
Call out "Help!" If someone comes, send that person to activate the EMS system.	This will summon emergency personnel while you continue to provide assistance to the child.
Do not perform blind finger sweep.	With loss of consciousness, object may be visible and removed. Blind finger sweeps should not be performed because they may push the obstructing object back into or further into the airway.
Open airway with head tilt–chin lift and try to give breaths. If the chest does not rise, reposition the head and try again to give rescue breaths.	Airway obstruction may be caused, in part, by improper head position.

Performance Guidelines

	Objectives
	Action: If airway is obstructed, perform Heimlich maneuver (up to 5 thrusts).
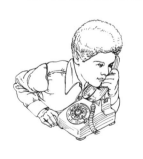	**Action:** Activate the EMS system after approximately 1 minute.

Critical Performance	Reason
Kneel astride the child's thighs or next to the thighs. Place the heel of one hand on the child's abdomen, in the midline, slightly above the navel but below the breastbone and xiphoid. Place the second hand on top of the first. Press into the abdomen with quick upward thrusts. • After 5 abdominal thrusts, open the airway with a tongue-jaw lift and remove the object if you see it. • Try to give 2 rescue breaths. • If unsuccessful, reposition the head and reattempt breaths. • If still unsuccessful, perform 5 more abdominal thrusts. Repeat this sequence until rescue breaths are successful.	Such thrusts may expel the object.
If you are alone, activate the EMS system after approximately 1 minute of effort.	

Performance Guidelines

Relief of Obstructed Airway: Child Becomes Unconscious (continued)

	Objectives
	Action: When obstruction is removed, check for breathing and pulse.

Critical Performance	Reason
Open the airway and check for breathing. • If there is no breathing, give 2 breaths. Check for a pulse. — If a pulse is present, provide 20 breaths per minute and continue to monitor pulse. — If there is no pulse, begin cycles of compressions and breaths. • If breathing resumes and there is no evidence of trauma, place the child on one side in the recovery position and await the arrival of emergency personnel.	

Performance Guidelines

Relief of Obstructed Airway: Unconscious Child (1 to 8 years)

	Objectives
	Assessment: Determine unre-sponsiveness. Shout for help.
	Action: Position the child on back.
	Action: Open the airway. **Assessment:** Determine breathlessness.

Critical Performance	Reason
Tap or gently shake victim's shoulder. Shout "Are you OK?" Call out "Help!"	This initial call for help is to alert bystanders so they can activate the EMS system while you care for the child.
Turn child on back holding head and body as a unit, supporting head and neck.	
Use the head tilt–chin lift maneuver to position the child's head in a neutral position and open the airway.	
Place your ear over the child's mouth and observe the chest. *Look* at the chest for movement. *Listen* for the sounds of breathing. *Feel* for breath on your cheek.	You must determine that the child is not breathing.

Performance Guidelines

Relief of Obstructed Airway: Unconscious Child (1 to 8 years) (continued)

	Objectives
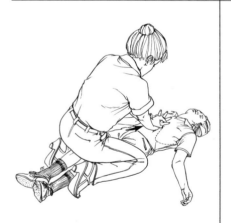	**Action:** Open the airway and try to give 2 rescue breaths. Observe the rise of the chest with each breath. **Action:** If initial rescue breaths are unsuccessful, reposition the head and try again. If repeat attempts are unsuccessful, perform Heimlich thrusts.
	Action: Perform the Heimlich maneuver (up to 5 thrusts).

Critical Performance	Reason
Use the thumb and forefinger of the hand that is maintaining pressure on the child's forehead to pinch the nostrils closed. Make a tight seal with your mouth over the child's mouth. Give 2 rescue breaths.	Complete airway obstruction by a foreign body is assumed if the child becomes unconscious, but if the child is found unconscious, an attempt must be made to get some air into the lungs. If the chest rises, the airway is open. If the chest does not rise, the airway is obstructed.
Reposition the child's head and lift the chin. Pinch the nostrils closed. Seal the mouth properly and try again to give rescue breaths.	Improper head tilt–chin lift is the most common reason that airway obstruction is not relieved.
The Heimlich maneuver: Kneel at the child's hips if the child is on the floor; stand at child's side if the child is on a table. If the child is large, you may kneel astride the child's thighs. Place the heel of one hand on the abdomen midline, slightly above the navel and well below the sternum and xiphoid. Place the second hand directly on top of the first hand. Press into the abdomen with quick upward thrusts.	Such thrusts can force air upward into the airway from the lungs with enough pressure to expel the foreign body.

Performance Guidelines

	Objectives
	Action: Perform tongue-jaw lift. Check for a foreign object and if you see it, remove it.
	Action: Open the airway and try to give rescue breaths. If unsuccessful, reposition the head and try again.

Critical Performance	Reason
Lift tongue and jaw forward by putting your thumb in the child's mouth over the tongue and wrapping your fingers around the lower jaw. If you see a foreign body, remove it. *Do not* perform a blind finger sweep.	A dislodged foreign body may now be manually accessible if it has not been expelled. Blind finger sweeps may push the obstructing object back into or further into the airway.
Position the child's head using the head tilt–chin lift maneuver. Seal the mouth properly and try again to give rescue breaths. If the airway remains obstructed, alternate the following maneuvers in rapid sequence: • Perform Heimlich maneuver. • Perform tongue-jaw lift, check for foreign body, and remove it if seen. • Open the airway. • Attempt, reattempt rescue breathing while maintaining an open airway. Repeat this sequence until successful.	By this time another attempt must be made to get some air into the victim's lungs. You must try again to dislodge the foreign body and give rescue breaths. Persistent attempts should be made in sequence to relieve the obstruction. As the child becomes more deprived of oxygen, the muscles will relax, and maneuvers that were previously ineffective may become effective.

Performance Guidelines

Relief of Obstructed Airway: Unconscious Child (1 to 8 years) (continued)

	Objectives
	Action: Activate the EMS system after approximately 1 minute.

Critical Performance	Reason

If you are alone, activate the EMS system after approximately 1 minute of effort.
 	
• If there is no breathing, give 2 breaths. Check for a pulse.
  — If a pulse is present, provide 20 breaths per minute and continue to monitor pulse.
  — If there is no pulse, begin cycles of compressions and breaths.
• If breathing resumes and there is no evidence of trauma, place the child on one side in the recovery position and await the arrival of emergency personnel.	

Appendix A
Skill Performance Sheets

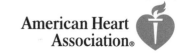

American Heart Association®

Fighting Heart Disease and Stroke

Student Name _____ Date _____

Child One-Rescuer CPR

Performance Guidelines	Performed
1. Establish unresponsiveness. If second rescuer is available, have him or her activate the EMS system.	
2. Open airway (head tilt–chin lift or jaw thrust). Check breathing (look, listen, feel).*	
3. Give 2 slow breaths (1 to 1½ seconds per breath), watch chest rise, allow for exhalation between breaths.	
4. Check carotid pulse. If breathing is absent but pulse is present, provide rescue breathing (1 breath every 3 seconds, about 20 breaths per minute).	
5. If no pulse, give 5 chest compressions (100 compressions per minute), open airway, and provide 1 slow breath. Repeat this cycle.	
6. After about 1 minute of rescue support, check pulse.* If rescuer is alone, activate the EMS system. If no pulse, continue 5:1 cycles.	

*If victim is breathing or resumes effective breathing, place in recovery position.

Comments _____

_____

_____

Instructor _____

Circle one: Complete   Needs more practice

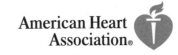

American Heart
Association®

Fighting Heart Disease and Stroke

Student Name _____ Date _____

Child Foreign-Body Airway Obstruction — Conscious

Performance Guidelines	Performed
1. Ask "Are you choking?"	
2. Give abdominal thrusts.	
3. Repeat thrusts until effective or victim becomes unconscious.	
Child Foreign-Body Airway Obstruction — Victim Becomes Unconscious	
4. If second rescuer is available, have him or her activate the EMS system.	
5. Perform a tongue-jaw lift, and if you see the object, perform a finger sweep to remove it.	
6. Open airway and try to ventilate; if still obstructed, reposition head and try to ventilate again.	
7. Give up to 5 abdominal thrusts.	
8. Repeat steps 5 through 7 until effective.*	
9. If airway obstruction is not relieved after about 1 minute, activate the EMS system.	

*If victim is breathing or resumes effective breathing, place in recovery position.

Comments _____

_____

_____

Instructor _____

Circle one: Complete   Needs more practice

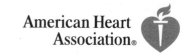

American Heart
Association®

Fighting Heart Disease and Stroke

Student Name _____ Date _____

Child Foreign-Body Airway Obstruction — Unconscious

Performance Guidelines	Performed
1. Establish unresponsiveness. If second rescuer is available, have him or her activate the EMS system.	
2. Open airway and try to ventilate; if still obstructed, reposition head and try to ventilate again.	
3. Give up to 5 abdominal thrusts.	
4. Perform a tongue-jaw lift, and if you see the object, perform a finger sweep to remove it.	
5. Repeat steps 2 through 4 until effective.*	
6. If airway obstruction is not relieved after about 1 minute, activate the EMS system.	

*If victim is breathing or resumes effective breathing, place in recovery position.

Comments _____

_____

_____

Instructor _____

Circle one: Complete   Needs more practice

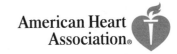

American Heart Association®

Fighting Heart Disease and Stroke

Student Name _____ Date _____

Infant One-Rescuer CPR

Performance Guidelines	Performed
1. Establish unresponsiveness. If second rescuer is available, have him or her activate the EMS system.	
2. Open airway (head tilt–chin lift or jaw thrust). Check breathing (look, listen, feel).*	
3. Give 2 slow breaths (1 to 1½ seconds per breath), watch chest rise, allow for exhalation between breaths.	
4. Check brachial pulse. If breathing is absent but pulse is present, provide rescue breathing (1 breath every 3 seconds, about 20 breaths per minute).	
5. If no pulse, give cycles of 5 chest compressions (rate, at least 100 compressions per minute) followed by 1 slow breath.	
6. After about 1 minute of rescue support, check pulse.* If rescuer is alone, activate the EMS system. If no pulse, continue 5:1 cycles.	

*If victim is breathing or resumes effective breathing, place in recovery position.

Comments _____

_____

_____

Instructor _____ ___

Circle one: Complete   Needs more practice

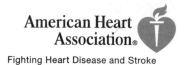

Student Name _____ Date _____

Infant Foreign-Body Airway Obstruction — Conscious

Performance Guidelines	Performed
1. Confirm complete airway obstruction. Check for serious breathing difficulty, ineffective cough, *no* strong cry.	
2. Give up to 5 back blows and 5 chest thrusts.	
3. Repeat step 2 until effective or victim becomes unconscious.	
Infant Foreign-Body Airway Obstruction — Victim Becomes Unconscious	
4. If second rescuer is available, have him or her activate the EMS system.	
5. Perform a tongue-jaw lift, and if you see the object, perform a finger sweep to remove it.	
6. Open airway and try to ventilate; if still obstructed, reposition head and try to ventilate again.	
7. Give up to 5 back blows and 5 chest thrusts.	
8. Repeat steps 5 through 7 until effective.*	
9. If airway obstruction is not relieved after about 1 minute, activate the EMS system.	

*If victim is breathing or resumes effective breathing, place in recovery position.

Comments _____

_____

_____

Instructor _____

Circle one: Complete   Needs more practice

Appendix A
Skill Performance Sheets

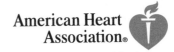

American Heart
Association®

Fighting Heart Disease and Stroke

Student Name _____ Date _____

Infant Foreign-Body Airway Obstruction — Unconscious

Performance Guidelines	Performed
1. Establish unresponsiveness. If second rescuer is available, have him or her activate the EMS system.	
2. Open airway and try to ventilate; if still obstructed, reposition head and try to ventilate again.	
3. Give up to 5 back blows and 5 chest thrusts.	
4. Perform a tongue-jaw lift, and if you see the object, perform a finger sweep to remove it.	
5. Repeat steps 2 through 4 until effective.*	
6. If airway obstruction is not relieved after about 1 minute, activate the EMS system.	

*If victim is breathing or resumes effective breathing, place in recovery position.

Comments _____

_____

_____

Instructor _____

Circle one: Complete   Needs more practice

Appendix B
Checklist

This checklist is an important part of this program. Take it with you on an inspection tour of your home, day-care center, school, baby-sitter's home, or wherever a child spends time.

Circle your answers to the various questions and check the appropriate box when the installation of a safety item is indicated. We recommend that you pair up with a classmate if possible and conduct an inspection tour together in your homes or child-care facility. The tour takes about 1 hour.

If you circle the answer printed in the first column, steps have been taken to help ensure a safe environment for children.

If you circle the answer in the column headed "Unsafe," some changes need to be made. If you are inspecting your own home or a child-care facility in which you work, consider making the changes immediately. If you are inspecting a day-care facility designed for the care of children away from home, speak with the director or other person in charge of the facility about the importance of safety. Show the director the checklist and, if possible, tour the facility with him or her.

The fourth column is designed for you to indicate that the purchase and installation of a safety item is recommended. Make sure the item is installed as soon as possible. You may want to arrange for another safety tour to be sure the recommended changes have been made.

If your inspection tour prevents even one injury, it will have been well worth your time and effort.

Checklist

Car Safety	Safe	Unsafe	Not Applicable	Purchase Safety Item
1. Do you and every person who rides with you buckle up during all auto travel?	Yes	No		
2. Do children 12 years old or younger ride in the BACK seat with appropriate child safety seat or lap-shoulder restraints?	Yes	No		
3. If you are using a safety seat made for infants only, does it always face backward? Is it always secured in the BACK seat of the car? (NEVER place a rear-facing infant seat in the front seat of a car with a passenger-side air bag.)	Yes	No	NA	
4. If you are using a convertible seat, do you follow the manu-facturer's instructions for con-verting it from infant to toddler use? (Be sure to wait until the child weighs at least 20 pounds or is older than 1 year and can sit well alone before using the forward-facing position.) Do you always place this seat in the BACK seat of the car?	Yes	No	NA	
5. If you are using a seat made for toddlers, is it . . .			NA	
Used only for children who weigh at least 20 pounds or are older than 1 year?	Yes	No		
Always used in the forward-facing position?	Yes	No		
Always used to secure the toddler in the BACK seat of the car?		Yes	No	
6. If a child safety seat is being used, is the . . .			NA	
Child large enough (at least 30 pounds)?	Yes	No		

Car Safety (Cont.)	Safe	Unsafe	Not Applicable	Purchase Safety Item
Three-point seat belt (with lap and shoulder belt) used when appropriate?	Yes	No		
Shield (if provided) fastened very close to the child's body?	Yes	No		
Tethered harness (if required) properly installed?	Yes	No		
Child safety seat always used to secure the child in the BACK seat of the car?		Yes	No	
7. Is the child properly secured in the child safety seat (all types)? Is the. . .			NA	
Harness over the shoulders and snug?	Yes	No		
Crotch strap taut (not loose)?	Yes	No		
Shield (if provided) close to the child's body and used with the harness?	Yes	No		
Tether strap (if required) installed properly?	Yes	No		
Child safety seat properly located in the BACK seat of the car?		Yes	No	
8. Is the seat/lap belt in the correct place and tight? Did you . . .				
Place the belt in the correct route? (Follow the instructions for the seat you are using. Don't guess. Each model is different. The belt may go through the seat frame, through a slot in the shell, or over the child's lap.)	Yes	No		
Test for tightness by pushing the seat forward and backward? (It should not move. If it does, tighten the belt while pressing the safety seat firmly into the auto seat cushion with your knee. If the belt has a wind-up reel, feed the webbing back into it to take up all the slack. If the safety belt remains loose or	Yes	No		

Car Safety (Cont.)	Safe	Unsafe	Not Applicable	Purchase Safety Item
loosens when the seat is pushed hard, check the placement of the buckle. For proper adjustment, the buckle and latchplate must be located well below the frame or toward the center of the seat. If the buckle or latchplate lies just at the point where the belt must bend around the frame or through the slot of the safety seat, the belt cannot be tightened properly. If this belt must be used, shorten the buckle end by twisting the webbing of the buckle several times so the latchplate will lie well below the bend. Look for another set of belts in the car that can be tightened properly. The center rear belt can usually be tightened by hand. The lap-shoulder belt can be kept snug by adding a locking clip.) **Note:** Car safety seats that are convertible (fitting from birth to about 40 pounds) usually have different belt routes for use when facing forward and backward. Use the appropriate one.				
9. Is the child ready for a regular safety belt? Does he or she . . . Use a combination lap-shoulder belt, which provides better protection than a lap belt alone? (The shoulder belt should fit across the shoulder. Be sure that the lap belt rests low across the child's hips and that the shoulder belt crosses from hip to shoulder, not across the neck. For children 4 to 7 years old, child safety seats may be needed to restrain the child properly with a lap-shoulder restraint system.)	Yes	No	NA	

General Indoor Safety	Safe	Unsafe	Not Applicable	Purchase Safety Item
Use a lap belt, if that is the only belt available? (It must be worn tight and across the hips, not across the stomach. The back seat is best for lap-belt use.)	Yes	No		
SIT properly restrained in the BACK seat?	Yes	No		
10. Is a sticker with emergency telephone numbers on the telephone? (It must include the telephone numbers for the EMS system, police, fire department, local hospital or physician, the poison control center in your area, and your telephone number.)	Yes	No		
11. Are working smoke detectors properly placed? Are they . . .				
On the ceiling or 6 to 12 inches below the ceiling?	Yes	No		
In the hallway outside sleeping or napping areas?	Yes	No		
On each floor at head of stairs to basement and at head of stairs to bedrooms?	Yes	No		
Tested monthly and batteries replaced twice every year when the clocks are changed to and from daylight saving time?	Yes	No		
12. Are there two unobstructed exits from the home, child-care facility, classroom, etc? (These are vital in case of fire or other emergency.)	Yes	No		
13. Has a fire escape plan been developed and practiced?	Yes	No		
14. Does each child know how to "stop, drop, and roll" to put out flames if his or her clothes catch on fire?	Yes	No		

General Indoor Safety (Cont.)	Safe	Unsafe	Not Applicable	Purchase Safety Item
15. Is there a working fire extinguisher (to put out a small fire or to clear an escape path)?	Yes	No		
16. Are all space heaters approved, in safe condition, and out of a child's reach? (Each space heater should be stable, have a protective covering, and be placed at least 3 feet from curtains, papers, and furniture.)	Yes	No		
17. Are all wood-burning stoves safe and out of a child's reach and vented properly? Are they . . .			NA	
Inspected yearly (including chimneys and stovepipes)?	Yes	No		
Behind a protective screen?	Yes	No		
18. Are electric cords (extension and appliance cords) in safe condition — not frayed or overloaded?	Yes	No		
19. Wherever practical, are electric cords placed out of a child's reach? (Children sucking or biting on live electric cords can receive severe electric burns.)	Yes	No		
20. Are shock stops (plastic outlet plugs) or outlet covers installed on all electric outlets? (These can keep a child from sticking an object into an exposed outlet or sucking on an exposed extension cord outlet.)	Yes	No		
21. Do you or the caregiver always keep one hand on the infant while he or she is on a high surface such as a changing table?	Yes	No	NA	

General Indoor Safety (Cont.)	Safe	Unsafe	Not Applicable	Purchase Safety Item
22. Is the crib safe? Does the . . .			NA	
Crib mattress fit snugly, with no more than the distance of two fingers between mattress and crib railing? (A child's head may become caught between a loose-fitting mattress and a bed frame.)	Yes	No		
Distance between crib slats measures 2⅜ inches or less? (A child can be caught or strangled between bars that are more than 2⅜ inches apart.)	Yes	No		
23. Are stairs, railings, porches, and balconies sturdy and in good condition?	Yes	No	NA	
24. Is hall and stairway lighting adequate to prevent falls?	Yes	No	NA	
25. Are toddler gates used at the top and bottom of stairs? (Accordion-type gates with wide spaces at the top should not be used. They can entrap a child's head and cause strangulation.)	Yes	No	NA	
26. Does your child use an infant walker?	No	Yes		Eliminate walker.
27. Are windows above the ground floor secure so that a child can't fall out?	Yes	No	NA	

General Indoor Safety (Cont.)	Safe	Unsafe	Not Applicable	Purchase Safety Item
28. Is syrup of ipecac kept on hand in case of a poisoning? (Parents should keep one bottle of ipecac in the home for each young child in their care; two or three bottles should be enough for the initial dose for 4 to 5 children. Like other medications, ipecac should be kept beyond the reach of children. Syrup of ipecac should be given only under the direction of a poison control center or a physician.)	Yes	No		
29. Are medicine and vitamins stored beyond the reach of children and in child-resistant packages? (Children like to imitate adults "taking medicine.")	Yes	No		
30. Are cleaning supplies stored out of the reach and sight of a child? Do you . . . Store all household poisons in original containers in high places, not under the kitchen sink? (The best storage place for poisons is a high, locked cabinet or closet.)	Yes	No		
Store cleaning supplies separately from food?	Yes	No		
31. Are safety latches or locks installed on cabinets that contain potentially dangerous items and are within the reach of a child? (For example, cleaning supplies, medicine, alcohol, knives, firearms, matches, and tools should be locked well away from children.)	Yes	No		

General Indoor Safety (Cont.)

	Safe	Unsafe	Not Applicable	Purchase Safety Item
32. Are purses with vitamins, medications, cigarettes, matches, jewelry, and calculators (with easy-to-swallow button batteries) kept out of children's reach?	Yes	No		
33. Can children get into the basement or garage, where dangerous products are often stored? (A hook-and-eye latch should be placed 5 feet or higher above the bottom of the door.)	No	Yes	NA	
34. Are potentially harmful plants out of a child's reach? (Many plants are poisonous. Consult your poison control center.)	Yes	No	NA	
35. Is there any loose, chipping, or peeling paint on walls or furniture? (Children can be poisoned by lead paint. If there is any suspicion, have the child tested for lead poisoning.)	No	Yes		
36. Do toy chests have lightweight lids, no lids, or safe-closing hinges? (A dropping lid can cause suffocation or head and neck injuries.)	Yes	No	NA	

Kitchen Safety

	Safe	Unsafe		
37. Are coffee, other hot liquids, and hot foods placed out of the reach of a child? Do you and the caregiver . . .				
Carry a child while holding hot liquids or food? (Carry hot items separately — make two trips!)	No	Yes		
Place hot liquids and food away from the table's edge?	Yes	No		

Kitchen Safety (Cont.)	Safe	Unsafe	Not Applicable	Purchase Safety Item
Avoid tablecloths and placemats that can be yanked down, spilling hot liquids or food?	Yes	No		
Keep children in a safe place while you are cooking?	Yes	No		
Cook on the back stove burners when possible and turn pot handles to the inside?	Yes	No		
Keep high chairs and stools away from the stove?	Yes	No		
Keep food treats and other attractive items next to or over the stove?	No	Yes		
Test the temperature of heated food before feeding children?	Yes	No		
Teach young children the meaning of the word *hot*?	Yes	No		
38. Are foods and small items (including balloons) that can choke a child kept out of reach?	Yes	No		
39. Are knives and other sharp objects kept out of the reach of children?	Yes	No		

Bathroom Safety

	Safe	Unsafe	Not Applicable	Purchase Safety Item
40. Are infants and young children always watched by an adult while in the tub? (Children can drown in a few inches of water within minutes. They can be burned by turning on the hot water themselves.)	Yes	No		
41. Are skidproof mats or stickers used in the bathtub?	Yes	No		
42. Is the water heat adjusted to a safe temperature? (A setting of 120°F or less prevents tap water scalds in sinks as well as in tubs.) Hot water temperature: _____°F. (Let the water run for 3 minutes before testing it.)	Yes	No		

Bathroom Safety (Cont.)	Safe	Unsafe	Not Applicable	Purchase Safety Item
43. Are electric appliances (radios, hair dryers, space heaters, etc) kept out of the bathroom or unplugged, away from water, and beyond the reach of a child? (These appliances can cause serious electric shock or death if they are plugged in and fall into a tub while the child is in the water or fall into a sink a child is using.)	Yes	No		

Firearms

	Safe	Unsafe	Not Applicable	Purchase Safety Item
44. Are firearms present in the home?	No	Yes		
Are they stored . . .			NA	
Inaccessible to children and adolescents in the home?	Yes	No		
Unloaded and separate from ammunition?	Yes	No		
Locked with a trigger lock or in a lockbox?	Yes	No		Trigger lock

Outdoor Safety

	Safe	Unsafe	Not Applicable	Purchase Safety Item
45. Is playground equipment safe? Is the equipment . . .			NA	
Assembled correctly according to manufacturer's instructions?	Yes	No		
Anchored properly over a level, soft surface, such as sand or wood chips?	Yes	No		
46. Is the child ready for safe bicycling? Does the child . . .			NA	
Ride on the right-sized bicycle on the right side of the road?	Yes	No		
Wear a protective helmet?	Yes	No		
Ride double or on a borrowed or unfamiliar bike?	No	Yes		

Outdoor Safety (Cont.)	Safe	Unsafe	Not Applicable	Purchase Safety Item
47. Do you allow children to play with fireworks?	No	Yes		
48. Is the child properly protected while roller skating or skate-boarding? Does the child . . .			NA	
Wear a helmet and protective padding for knees and elbows?	Yes	No		
Skate in rinks or parks that are free of traffic?	Yes	No		
Perform daredevil and stunt riding techniques?	No	Yes		
49. Is the child properly protected while riding on sleds or snowdisks? Does the child . . .			NA	
Use a sturdy sled with a good steering mechanism and no sharp edges?	Yes	No		
Sled only in daylight and in a safe, supervised area away from motor vehicles?	Yes	No		
Ever sled on an ice pond?	No	Yes		
Know how to steer and stop the sled?	Yes	No		
50. Is the child properly protected while participating in contact sports? Do you . . .			NA	
Provide proper adult instruction and supervision?	Yes	No		
Place children together with others of similar weight and size?	Yes	No		
Always have the child wear appropriate safety equipment (eye shields, helmets, mouth guards, athletic cups, etc)?	Yes	No		

Outdoor Safety (Cont.)	Safe	Unsafe	Not Applicable	Purchase Safety Item
51. Is the child properly protected from animal bites? Do you . . .				
Refrain from having a pet until the child is old enough (around 6 years old) to understand how to treat an animal?	Yes	No		
Teach the child how to handle and care for a pet?	Yes	No		
Teach the child to avoid strange animals, especially wild, sick, or injured ones?	Yes	No		
Teach the child never to break up an animal fight, even when a familiar pet is involved?	Yes	No		
Stress the importance of avoiding bicycle routes where dogs are known to chase vehicles?	Yes	No		
Alert the child to dangerous or nervous animals in the area and teach him or her to avoid entering yards or houses that harbor them?	Yes	No		
52. Do you have a home swimming pool and children 5 years of age or younger?	No	Yes		
Are children *always* supervised by an adult during swimming?	Yes	No	NA	
Is the pool totally enclosed with fencing 4 to 5 feet high or higher?	Yes	No	NA	
Are all gates self-closing and self-latching?	Yes	No	NA	
Do you change young children from swimsuits into street clothes and remove all toys from the pool area at the end of swim time?	Yes	No	NA	
Does every member of the family 12 years of age or older know CPR?	Yes	No		

Outdoor Safety (Cont.)	Safe	Unsafe	Not Applicable	Purchase Safety Item
53. Are pools on nearby properties protected from use by unsupervised children?	Yes	No	NA	
54. Is the child ready for safe swimming? (Never permit a child to swim alone or unsupervised.)	Yes	No		

Note: Much of the safety information presented in this course is based on the SAFEHOME program developed by the Massachusetts Department of Public Health as part of its Statewide Comprehensive Injury Prevention Program and the Children's Traffic Safety Program at Vanderbilt University in Nashville. The SAFEHOME program was funded by the Federal Division of Maternal and Child Health. The Children's Traffic Safety Program was funded by the Department of Transportation and the Tennessee Governor's Highway Safety Program.

Appendix C
Self-test Questions

1. **The most common cause of cardiac arrest in infants and children is:**

   a. heart attack

   b. respiratory arrest or breathing problem

   c. electric shock

   d. congenital heart abnormality

   Answer, p. 27

2. **It is important to know about the risk factors for heart disease because:**

   a. they indicate whether you are going to have a heart attack

   b. it may be possible to reduce the risk of heart disease through a healthy lifestyle

   c. they scare people into quitting smoking

   d. they can help you recover from a heart attack

   Answer, p. 18

3. **Before the rescuer attempts to resuscitate a victim by providing rescue breathing, the following condition should exist:**

   a. brain damage

   b. dilated pupils

   c. absence of breathing

   d. effective respirations

   Answer, pp. 34-35, 42-43

4. The most common cause of airway obstruction in the _unconscious_ victim is:

a. food

b. tongue

c. mucus

d. dentures

Answer, p. 28

5. Before CPR is begun, the rescuer should first:

a. examine the victim's mouth for foreign bodies

b. determine unresponsiveness

c. perform the Heimlich maneuver

d. open the airway

Answer, pp. 34, 42

6. If the airway seems obstructed after the initial attempt to ventilate an unconscious patient, the rescuer should:

a. reposition the head and attempt ventilation again

b. begin chest compressions

c. go on to check the pulse

d. check for foreign-body airway obstruction

Answer, pp. 56, 75

7. The principal method used for opening the airway when trauma is not a suspected cause of injury is:

a. head tilt with chin lift

b. turning the head to one side

c. striking the victim on the back

d. wiping out the mouth and throat

Answer, p. 28, 43

8. **The presence of breathing in an unconscious victim can be determined by:**

   a. checking for pupil dilation

   b. checking for discoloration of skin

   c. checking the pulse

   d. looking, listening, and feeling for air exchange

   Answer, pp. 43, 63, 81

9. **If breathing does not seem to be present after opening the airway:**

   a. begin chest compressions

   b. determine pulselessness

   c. check pupils

   d. give two rescue breaths

   Answer, pp. 36, 44

10. **When the rescuer is alone with a child who is a cardiac arrest victim and there is no possibility that another person will arrive, the rescuer should:**

    a. activate the EMS system before opening the victim's airway

    b. do nothing and wait for help to arrive

    c. open the victim's airway, then activate the EMS system

    d. perform CPR for 1 minute, then activate the EMS system

    Answer, p. 50

11. **If a choking victim is coughing forcefully:**

    a. check the pulse

    b. perform the Heimlich maneuver 5 times

    c. sweep out the mouth

    d. do not interfere

    Answer, p. 31

12. **In infants and children, the ratio of compressions to ventilations is:**

   a. 15 compressions to 2 ventilations

   b. 15 compressions to 5 ventilations

   c. 5 compressions to 2 ventilations

   d. 5 compressions to 1 ventilation

   Answer, pp. 40, 50

13. **All of the following are risk factors of heart disease except:**

   a. cigarette smoking

   b. high-fat, high-cholesterol diet

   c. high blood pressure

   d. nausea and vomiting

   Answer, p. 18

14. **After the rescuer provides back blows, if the airway of a 1-month-old infant is still obstructed (ventilation is not successful):**

   a. perform the Heimlich maneuver 5 times

   b. give 5 additional back blows

   c. give 5 chest thrusts

   d. turn the infant upside down and shake him or her

   Answer, p. 58

15. **To determine if there is an obstructed airway in a *conscious* child, the rescuer should:**

   a. ask the victim, "Are you choking?"

   b. shake the victim

   c. reposition the victim

   d. perform the Heimlich maneuver 5 times

   Answer, p. 31

16. Syrup of ipecac should be given:

a. only on the advice of a physician or poison control center

b. only to children over age 3

c. any time you suspect a child has swallowed a poisonous substance

d. any time you know a child has swallowed a poisonous substance

Answer, p. 12

17. The best place to store poisonous substances is:

a. on a high shelf

b. in a high, locked cabinet

c. in a garage

d. under a sink

Answer, p. 13

18. You can help prevent scalding burns by:

a. cooking on the back burners of a stove

b. turning pot handles inward on the stove

c. turning down the temperature of the water heater to 120°F

d. all of the above

Answer, pp. 10, 102-103

19. The No. 1 preventable cause of death in young children is:

a. drowning

b. heart attack

c. injuries suffered while riding in cars

d. communicable diseases

Answer, p. 7

20. To help prevent injuries and deaths from fires, each home or day-care facility should have:

a. two exits

b. a smoke detector

c. a fire extinguisher

d. all of the above

Answer, pp. 10, 98-99

Answer questions 21 through 25 if your course includes information about CPR for *infants*.

21. According to guidelines of the American Heart Association, infant CPR techniques are recommended for victims up to approximately the age of:

a. 1 month

b. 6 months

c. 1 year

d. 8 years

Answer, p. 3

22. In performing CPR, compress the infant's chest:

a. as gently as possible

b. as forcefully as possible

c. with sufficient force to depress the sternum one third to one half the depth of the chest

d. exactly 2 inches

Answer, p. 39

23. The rate of chest compressions in an infant is at least:

a. 90 times per minute

b. 100 times per minute

c. 80 times per minute

d. 60 times per minute

Answer, p. 39

24. The rescuer should check the infant's pulse by feeling the:

a. carotid pulse in the neck

b. brachial pulse in the arm

c. radial pulse in the wrist

d. femoral pulse in the groin

Answer, pp. 36-37

25. When giving rescue breaths to an infant, make a tight seal between your mouth and the infant's:

a. nose

b. mouth

c. nose and mouth

d. none of the above

Answer, p. 37

Answer questions 26 through 30 if your course includes information about CPR for *children.*

26. According to guidelines of the American Heart Association, child CPR techniques are performed on a victim:

a. under 1 year of age

b. 1 to 8 years of age

c. 8 to 10 years of age

d. 10 to 12 years of age

Answer, p. 3

27. In performing CPR, compress the child's chest:

a. as gently as possible

b. as firmly as possible

c. with sufficient force to depress the sternum approximately one third to one half the depth of the chest

d. exactly 2 to 2½ inches

Answer, p. 49

28. The rate of chest compression in a child is:

a. 60 per minute

b. 60 to 80 per minute

c. 80 to 100 per minute

d. 100 per minute

Answer, p. 49

29. The rescuer should check the child's pulse by feeling the:

a. carotid pulse in the neck

b. brachial pulse in the arm

c. radial pulse in the wrist

d. femoral pulse in the groin

Answer, pp. 46-47

30. Rescue breathing for a child with a pulse should be performed:

a. 8 times per minute

b. 10 times per minute

c. 15 times per minute

d. 20 times per minute

Answer, p. 47

Appendix D
Legal and Ethical Issues

Recognition is given for successful completion of a CPR course, based on criteria established by the American Heart Association. Successful course completion does not imply licensure or warrant future performance.

There is no instance known in which a layperson who has performed CPR has been sued successfully. Good Samaritan laws in most states specifically protect professionals and laypersons performing CPR "in good faith." Under most Good Samaritan laws, laypersons are protected if they perform CPR even if they have had no formal training. All citizens should learn to perform CPR well enough to sustain the life of the victim until professional emergency medical treatment becomes available unless such performance would pose a medical or emotional danger to themselves.

As a rescuer acting in good faith, you should remember that once CPR is begun, you should stop only when one of the following occurs:

- The victim recovers (regains pulse and breathing).
- Another trained person takes over.
- You are too exhausted to continue.
- A valid DNR (Do-Not-Resuscitate) order is presented to the rescuer.

The Patient Self-determination Act of 1991 was intended to support the rights of patients to make decisions about their medical care and to make advance directives. Physicians and families should talk with patients about their preferences regarding CPR in various clinical settings. For more information, contact your physician or hospital.